MW01028688

LOW-FODMAP VEGETARIAN COOKBOOK

Healthy, Simple & Delicious Recipes
to Soothe your Gut, Manage
Digestive Disorders and Relieve IBS
with 4-Week meal plan

Dr. Mary D. Torres

Copyright 2023 by Dr. Mary D. Torres

All rights reserved.

This copyright applies to the entire contents of this cookbook, including but not limited to text, recipes, illustrations, photographs, and design. No part of this cookbook may be reproduced, distributed, or transmitted in any form or by any means, including photocopying, recording, or other electronic or mechanical methods, without the prior written permission of the copyright holder, except for brief quotations embodied in critical reviews and certain other non-commercial uses permitted by copyright law.

This book is a work of non-fiction. The recipes and advice provided herein are based on the author's personal experience, research, and expertise. Readers are advised to consult with healthcare professionals, nutritionists before making significant changes to their diet.

TABLE OF CONTENT

INTRODUCTION

Digestive issues, as we all know too well can cast a long shadow over daily life. Whether it's the agony of bloating, the discomfort of gas, or the anguish of abdominal pain, living with these symptoms can be frustrating. Gastrointestinal distress does not only affect physical well-being but can also leave a lasting impact on mental health and overall quality of life.

Ignoring the signs and symptoms that indicate a need for a Low-FODMAP diet can lead to more than just temporary discomfort. Chronic digestive issues can erode the quality of life, impacting energy levels, emotional well-being, and overall health. If left untreated, these issues can lead to more serious conditions, affecting not just physical health but also mental and emotional resilience.

This book is designed to be your trusted companion in embracing the low-FODMAP diet while staying true to your vegetarian or plant-based values. Whether you are already a vegetarian, considering adopting a plant-based diet, or just looking to explore a more digestive-friendly way of eating, this cookbook is tailored to meet your needs.

The Benefits of This Cookbook:

Digestive Comfort: This cookbook is designed to help you find freedom from the shackles of digestive discomfort. By understanding the Low-FODMAP diet, you'll be able to experience relief from bloating, gas, cramps, and other symptoms that may have plagued you for far too long.

Plant-Based and Palate-Pleasing: Going for a Low-FODMAP lifestyle doesn't mean sacrificing flavor. This cookbook is a testament to the fact that a plant-based diet can be both healthful and delicious. From hearty breakfasts to decadent desserts, each recipe is crafted with your palate in mind.

Comprehensive Guidance: Beyond recipes, this book provides in-depth guidance on navigating the Low-FODMAP lifestyle. You will learn step-by-step how to set up a Low-FODMAP food preparation, create balanced meals, and troubleshoot any challenges that may arise along the way.

Expertise and Trust: "The Low-FODMAP Vegetarian Cookbook" is the result of years of professional experience in the field of dietetics. You can trust that the information and recipes presented are grounded in sound nutritional science.

CHAPTER 1: BASICS OF LOW-FODMAP

What Are Fodmaps?

FODMAP is an acronym that stands for Fermentable Oligosaccharides, Disaccharides, Monosaccharides, and Polyols which is a group of fermentable, short-chain carbohydrates found in various foods. These compounds are known to be potential triggers for digestive discomfort and gastrointestinal symptoms in some individuals, particularly those with irritable bowel syndrome (IBS) and certain other gastrointestinal conditions.

Let's break down the components of FODMAP for better Understanding:

Fermentable: FODMAPs are carbohydrates that are readily fermented by the gut bacteria in the large intestine. This fermentation process produces gases, which can lead to bloating, gas, and abdominal discomfort.

Oligosaccharides: This category includes fructans and galacto-oligosaccharides (GOS). Foods high in fructans include wheat, rye, onions, and garlic, while GOS can be found in legumes and certain nuts.

Disaccharides: Lactose is a disaccharide sugar found in dairy products, falls into this category. Some people have difficulty digesting lactose, which often leads to symptoms like diarrhea and abdominal pain.

Monosaccharides: This category includes excess fructose, a type of sugar that can be problematic for some individuals. Foods high in excess fructose include honey, certain fruits like apples and pears, and high-fructose corn syrup.

Polyols: This is also known as sugar alcohols, polyols include compounds like sorbitol, mannitol, xylitol, and maltitol. These are often used as sweeteners in sugar-free and low-calorie products. Foods containing polyols include stone fruits (e.g., peaches and cherries) and artificial sweeteners.

For individuals who are sensitive to **FODMAPs,** consuming foods high in these carbohydrates can lead to a range of gastrointestinal symptoms, such as abdominal pain, bloating, gas, diarrhea, and constipation. The severity of these symptoms can vary from one person to another, and **FODMAP** intolerance is a common concern for those with IBS and other gastrointestinal conditions.

The **Low-FODMAP** diet, which restricts or limits the consumption of **high-FODMAP** foods has become an effective approach to managing these symptoms. By following this diet, individuals can identify their personal trigger foods, reduce gastrointestinal distress, and enjoy improved digestive comfort.

What is Low-FODMAP Diet?

A Low-FODMAP diet is a dietary approach designed to manage and alleviate the symptoms of gastrointestinal distress, primarily in individuals who have conditions like irritable bowel syndrome (IBS), inflammatory bowel disease (IBD), or other functional gastrointestinal disorders. The term **"FODMAP"** stands for Fermentable Oligosaccharides, Disaccharides, Monosaccharides, and Polyols, which are a group of fermentable carbohydrates found in various foods.

The primary goal of a **Low-FODMAP** diet is to reduce or limit the consumption of high-FODMAP foods, as these compounds can be poorly absorbed in the small intestine and may trigger digestive discomfort in some people. The specific categories of high-FODMAP foods include:

Oligosaccharides: These include fructans and galacto-oligosaccharides (GOS). Foods high in fructans include wheat, rye, onions, and garlic, while GOS can be found in legumes and certain nuts.

Disaccharides: Lactose, a disaccharide sugar found in dairy products, is a common high-FODMAP component.

Monosaccharides: This category includes excess fructose, a type of sugar. Foods high in excess fructose include honey, certain fruits like apples and pears, and high-fructose corn syrup.

Polyols: These are sugar alcohols like sorbitol, mannitol, xylitol, and maltitol. They are found in some fruits (e.g., peaches and cherries) and artificial sweeteners.

The Low-FODMAP diet typically involves two main phases:

Elimination Phase: During this phase, individuals reduce or eliminate high-FODMAP foods from their diet for a specified period, often several weeks. This aims to provide relief from digestive symptoms.

Reintroduction Phase: After the elimination phase, high-FODMAP foods are systematically reintroduced one at a time to identify which specific FODMAPs trigger symptoms in the individual. This phase helps to personalize the diet and allows people to enjoy a broader range of foods while avoiding only the specific FODMAPs that cause discomfort.

NOTE: It's important to emphasize that the Low-FODMAP diet is not intended as a long-term or permanent eating plan. The goal is to identify individual trigger foods and create a more tailored, sustainable diet that minimizes symptoms while maximizing dietary variety.

Foods to Avoid

When going on a **Low-FODMAP** diet, it's important to avoid or significantly limit foods that are high in FODMAPs, as these can trigger gastrointestinal discomfort. Below are a list of common high-FODMAP foods to avoid or reduce during the elimination phase of the diet:

Wheat-Based Products:

Bread, especially made from wheat or rye

Pasta made from wheat

Cereals containing wheat or barley

Baked goods with wheat flour

Certain Vegetables:

Onions

Garlic

Leeks

Shallots

Artichokes

Asparagus

Fruits High in Excess Fructose:

Apples

Pears

Watermelon

High-fructose corn syrup

Dairy Products High in Lactose:

Milk

Ice cream

Yogurt

Soft cheeses

Legumes High in GOS:

Lentils

Chickpeas

Certain beans (e.g., kidney beans)

Sweeteners and Artificial Sweeteners:

Honey

Agave syrup

High-fructose corn syrup

Sorbitol

Mannitol

Xylitol

Certain Fruits and Vegetables High in Polyols:

Stone fruits (e.g., peaches, cherries)

Avocado

Cauliflower

Mushrooms

Processed Foods with Hidden FODMAPs:

Processed foods often contain hidden sources of FODMAPs, such as onion or garlic powder, high-fructose corn syrup, or wheat-based additives. Careful label reading is essential.

Certain Sweeteners and Additives:

Sorbitol, mannitol, xylitol, and maltitol are sugar alcohols that should be avoided. These are often found in sugar-free gum, candies, and some processed foods.

The Role of FODMAPs in Digestive Discomfort

FODMAPs, which stands for Fermentable Oligosaccharides, Disaccharides, Monosaccharides, and Polyols play a significant role in digestive discomfort, particularly in individuals who are sensitive to these fermentable carbohydrates. Checkout how FODMAPs impact the digestive system and contribute to discomfort:

Fermentation in the Gut: When undigested FODMAPs reach the large intestine, they become a source of food for the natural bacteria residing there. As these bacteria ferment FODMAPs, they produce gases, such as hydrogen, methane, and carbon dioxide. The accumulation of these gases can lead to bloating and distension of the intestines, causing discomfort and a feeling of fullness.

Osmotic Effect: FODMAPs have an osmotic effect, meaning they draw water into the intestines. This increased water content can lead to diarrhea in some individuals, particularly those who are sensitive to specific types of FODMAPs.

Altered Gut Motility: FODMAPs can influence the contractions and movements of the digestive tract. For some people, this alteration in gut motility can result in symptoms like diarrhea, while in others, it might cause constipation.

Nerve Sensitivity: FODMAPs may trigger the nerves in the gut, leading to increased sensations of pain and discomfort. Individuals with conditions like irritable bowel syndrome (IBS) often have hypersensitive nerves in their gastrointestinal tract, making them more prone to experiencing discomfort in response to FODMAPs.

Interaction with Gut Immune System: In individuals with certain gut disorders, FODMAPs can interact with the immune system, leading to inflammation and exacerbating symptoms such as abdominal pain.

The Low-FODMAP diet helps by reducing the intake of these fermentable carbohydrates, helps alleviate the symptoms associated with their fermentation and osmotic effects. By carefully managing FODMAP intake, individuals can often experience significant relief from bloating, gas, abdominal pain, diarrhea, and constipation, thereby improving their overall quality of life and digestive well-being.

Benefits of a Low-FODMAP Vegetarian Diet

A Low-FODMAP vegetarian diet offers several significant benefits for individuals who experience gastrointestinal discomfort or have conditions like irritable bowel syndrome (IBS). Some of the benefits ae;

Reduced Digestive Discomfort: The primary benefit of a Low-FODMAP vegetarian diet is a significant reduction in digestive discomfort. It helps minimizing the intake of fermentable carbohydrates which help individuals experience relief from symptoms such as bloating, gas, abdominal pain, diarrhea, and constipation.

Improved Quality of Life: Gastrointestinal symptoms can significantly impact a person's quality of life. A Low-FODMAP diet can help individuals regain a sense of control over their digestive health, and allow them to enjoy meals without the fear of discomfort and embarrassment.

Enhanced Dietary Variety: Contrary to the misconception that a Low-FODMAP diet is overly restrictive, it encourages individuals to explore a wide range of low-FODMAP fruits, vegetables, grains, and other plant-based foods. This variety ensures a balanced and nutritious diet.

Sustainable Vegetarian Lifestyle: For individuals adopting a vegetarian lifestyle, a Low-FODMAP diet provides a roadmap to combine their dietary choices with digestive wellness. It offers the means to enjoy the benefits of both plant-based and low-FODMAP eating.

Personalized Nutrition: The Low-FODMAP diet is not a one-size-fits-all solution. It encourages a specific approach, which allows individuals to identify their specific FODMAP triggers. This knowledge empowers them to tailor their diet to their unique needs.

Potential Weight Management: For some, the reduction in gastrointestinal discomfort can lead to better appetite regulation and potential weight management. This can be especially relevant for those with IBS who experience fluctuations in appetite.

Better Nutrient Absorption: Reduced gastrointestinal distress can enhance nutrient absorption, this will help individuals get the most out of the food they consume. This can lead to improved overall health.

Long-Term Digestive Wellness: A well-executed Low-FODMAP diet can provide a foundation for long-term digestive wellness. Having identifying individual trigger foods, individuals can create a sustainable diet that minimizes discomfort while maximizing nutritional value.

Freedom to Enjoy Food: Perhaps the most significant benefit is the freedom to enjoy food without the looming threat of digestive symptoms. A well-managed Low-FODMAP diet allows individuals to savor meals, social gatherings, and the pleasures of eating without discomfort.

Key Principles of the Low-FODMAP Diet

The Low-FODMAP diet operates on several key principles aimed at managing gastrointestinal symptoms effectively. Some of the fundamental guidelines that form the foundation of this dietary approach include;

Identification of High-FODMAP Foods: The diet involves identifying foods high in Fermentable Oligosaccharides, Disaccharides, Monosaccharides, and Polyols (FODMAPs). This includes categories such as fructans (found in wheat, rye, garlic, and onions), lactose (found in dairy products), excess fructose (found in certain fruits and sweeteners), galacto-oligosaccharides (found in legumes), and polyols (found in some fruits and artificial sweeteners).

Elimination Phase: During the initial phase, individuals remove high-FODMAP foods from their diet for a specific period (usually 2-6 weeks). This elimination phase aims to provide relief from symptoms and establish a baseline.

Personalized Reintroduction: After the elimination phase, high-FODMAP foods are systematically reintroduced one at a time. This reintroduction phase helps identify specific FODMAPs that trigger symptoms in the individual, allowing for a more tailored approach to the diet.

Individualized Approach: The Low-FODMAP diet is highly individualized. What triggers symptoms in one person may not affect another. This specific approach ensures that the diet is tailored to the individual's specific sensitivities.

Portion Control: Some low-FODMAP foods can become high in FODMAPs when consumed in large quantities. Portion control is crucial to avoid exceeding individual tolerance levels.

Nutritional Balance: While avoiding high-FODMAP foods, it's essential to maintain a nutritionally balanced diet. This includes incorporating low-FODMAP sources of fiber, vitamins, and minerals to prevent nutritional deficiencies.

Regular Monitoring: Throughout the diet, individuals monitor their symptoms and food intake. Keeping a food diary can be particularly helpful in tracking the relationship between specific foods and symptoms.

Long-Term Maintenance: Once trigger foods are identified; individuals move into a long-term maintenance phase. In this phase, the diet is customized to include a wide variety of low-FODMAP foods that do not trigger symptoms, allowing for sustainable, symptom-free eating.

Flexibility and Adaptability: The Low-FODMAP diet is not meant to be overly restrictive in the long term. It's designed to provide a framework for managing symptoms. Individuals learn to adapt recipes and food choices to suit their dietary needs, enabling them to enjoy a diverse and satisfying diet.

CHAPTER 2: BREAKFAST RECIPES

1. Low-FODMAP Scrambled Tofu

Benefits: A protein-rich and savory breakfast to start your day.

Ingredients:

1 block of firm tofu, crumbled

1 tablespoon garlic-infused olive oil

1 cup diced bell peppers (red or yellow)

Fresh chives (green tops) for garnish

Salt and pepper to taste

Instructions:

In a skillet, heat the garlic-infused olive oil over medium heat.

Add diced bell peppers and sauté for a few minutes.

Add crumbled tofu and cook until heated through.

Season with salt and pepper.

Garnish with fresh chives and serve.

2. Low-FODMAP Omelette with Spinach

Benefits: A protein-packed and nutrient-rich breakfast option.

Ingredients:

3 eggs

1 cup fresh spinach

1 tablespoon garlic-infused olive oil

Lactose-free cheese (optional)

Salt and pepper to taste

Instructions:

In a bowl, whisk the eggs.

In a skillet, heat the garlic-infused olive oil over medium heat.

Pour the whisked eggs into the skillet.

Add fresh spinach and cheese (if desired).

Cook until the omelette is set.

Season with salt and pepper.

3. Low-FODMAP Breakfast Burrito

Benefits: A hearty and flavorful breakfast wrap that's easy on the stomach.

Ingredients:

Gluten-free tortilla or wrap

Scrambled eggs (using garlic-infused olive oil)

Diced bell peppers (red or yellow)

Sliced avocado

Salsa (ensure it's low-FODMAP)

Salt and pepper to taste

Instructions:

Warm the gluten-free tortilla or wrap.

Layer with scrambled eggs, diced bell peppers, sliced avocado, and salsa.

Season with salt and pepper.

Roll up the burrito and enjoy.

4. Low-FODMAP Chia Pudding

Benefits: A nutritious and filling breakfast that's kind to your digestive system.

Ingredients:

1/4 cup chia seeds

1 cup lactose-free almond milk (or suitable alternative)

1 tablespoon maple syrup (ensure it's low-FODMAP)

Fresh mixed berries (e.g., strawberries, blueberries)

A sprinkle of toasted coconut flakes (optional)

Instructions:

In a bowl, mix chia seeds, lactose-free almond milk, and maple syrup.

Stir well and let the mixture sit in the refrigerator for a few hours or overnight to thicken.

Serve the chia pudding topped with fresh mixed berries and a sprinkle of toasted coconut flakes if desired.

5. Low-FODMAP Frittata

Benefits: A versatile and nutrient-packed breakfast dish.

Ingredients:

6 eggs

1 cup fresh spinach

1 cup diced bell peppers (red or yellow)

1 cup diced zucchini, 1 tablespoon garlic-infused olive oil

Salt and pepper to taste

Instructions:

Preheat your oven to 350°F (175°C).

In an oven-safe skillet, heat the garlic-infused olive oil over medium heat.

Add diced bell peppers and zucchini, and sauté for a few minutes.

Whisk the eggs and pour them into the skillet.

Add fresh spinach.

Season with salt and pepper.

Transfer the skillet to the oven and bake for about 20-25 minutes or until the frittata is set.

6. Low-FODMAP Smoothie Bowl

Benefits: A refreshing and nutritious breakfast option.

Ingredients:

1 cup lactose-free yogurt (or suitable alternative)

1/2 cup fresh mixed berries (e.g., strawberries, blueberries)

1/2 banana (ripe but not overripe)

1 tablespoon chia seeds

A sprinkle of gluten-free granola

Fresh mint leaves for garnish

Instructions:

In a bowl, layer lactose-free yogurt, mixed berries, and banana slices.

Sprinkle with chia seeds and gluten-free granola.

Garnish with fresh mint leaves.

7. Low-FODMAP Peanut Butter Rice Cakes

Benefits: A quick and satisfying breakfast with a protein boost.

Ingredients:

Rice cakes (ensure they are low-FODMAP)

Natural peanut butter (no added sugar)

Sliced strawberries

A drizzle of maple syrup (ensure it's low-FODMAP)

Instructions:

Spread natural peanut butter on rice cakes.

Top with sliced strawberries.

Drizzle with a touch of maple syrup.

8. Low-FODMAP Green Smoothie

Benefits: A refreshing and nutrient-rich breakfast option.

Ingredients:

1 cup fresh spinach

1/2 cucumber (peeled and sliced)

1/2 banana (ripe but not overripe)

1 cup lactose-free almond milk (or suitable alternative)

1 tablespoon chia seeds

Instructions:

Blend fresh spinach, cucumber, banana, lactose-free almond milk, and chia seeds until smooth.

Serve as a green and nutritious smoothie.

9. Low-FODMAP Rice Porridge

Benefits: A comforting and gentle breakfast option.

Ingredients:

Cooked white rice (ensure it's low-FODMAP)

Lactose-free milk (e.g., almond milk)

Cinnamon and maple syrup (ensure they are low-FODMAP)

Sliced bananas (ripe but not overripe)

Instructions:

In a bowl, combine cooked rice and lactose-free milk.

Sprinkle with cinnamon and drizzle with maple syrup.

Top with sliced bananas.

10. Low-FODMAP Quinoa Breakfast Bowl

Benefits: A protein-rich and satisfying breakfast to kickstart your day.

Ingredients:

Cooked quinoa

Sliced strawberries

Sliced kiwi

A drizzle of maple syrup (ensure it's low-FODMAP)

Chopped nuts (e.g., almonds or walnuts)

Instructions:

In a bowl, layer cooked quinoa, sliced strawberries, and sliced kiwi.

Drizzle with a touch of maple syrup.

Sprinkle with chopped nuts.

11. Low-FODMAP Cheddar and Spinach Muffins

Benefits: A portable and savory breakfast option.

Ingredients:

1 cup gluten-free flour (ensure it's low-FODMAP)

1 cup lactose-free milk (e.g., almond milk)

1/2 cup shredded cheddar cheese

1/2 cup fresh spinach, chopped

1 egg, 1 tablespoon garlic-infused olive oil

1 teaspoon baking powder, Salt and pepper to taste

Instructions:

Preheat your oven to 350°F (175°C).

In a mixing bowl, combine gluten-free flour, baking powder, salt, and pepper.

In another bowl, whisk together lactose-free milk, egg, and garlic-infused olive oil.

Add the wet ingredients to the dry ingredients and mix until just combined.

Fold in shredded cheddar cheese and chopped spinach.

Spoon the mixture into muffin cups and bake for about 20-25 minutes or until they are cooked through.

12. Low-FODMAP Berry Pancakes

Benefits: A sweet and satisfying breakfast with digestive comfort in mind.

Ingredients:

1 cup gluten-free pancake mix (ensure it's low-FODMAP)

1/2 cup lactose-free milk (e.g., almond milk)

1/2 cup fresh mixed berries (e.g., strawberries, blueberries)

1 tablespoon maple syrup (ensure it's low-FODMAP)

Instructions:

In a bowl, prepare the pancake mix according to the package instructions, using lactose-free milk.

Fold in fresh mixed berries.

Cook the pancakes on a griddle.

Serve with a drizzle of maple syrup.

13. Low-FODMAP Greek Yogurt Parfait

Benefits: A creamy and balanced breakfast that's easy on the stomach.

Ingredients:

1 cup lactose-free Greek yogurt

1/2 cup fresh mixed berries (e.g., strawberries, blueberries)

1 tablespoon maple syrup (ensure it's low-FODMAP)

A sprinkle of gluten-free granola

Instructions:

In a glass, layer lactose-free Greek yogurt, fresh mixed berries, and gluten-free granola.

Drizzle with a touch of maple syrup.

14. Low-FODMAP Zucchini and Feta Muffins

Benefits: A savory and portable breakfast option.

Ingredients:

1 cup grated zucchini, 1/2 cup crumbled feta cheese

1 cup gluten-free flour (ensure it's low-FODMAP)

1/2 cup lactose-free milk (e.g., almond milk)

1 egg, 1 tablespoon garlic-infused olive oil

1 teaspoon baking powder

Salt and pepper to taste

Instructions:

Preheat your oven to 350°F (175°C).

Place the grated zucchini in a clean kitchen towel and squeeze out excess moisture.

In a mixing bowl, combine gluten-free flour, baking powder, salt, and pepper.

In another bowl, whisk together lactose-free milk, egg, and garlic-infused olive oil.

Add the wet ingredients to the dry ingredients and mix until just combined.

Fold in grated zucchini and crumbled feta cheese.

Spoon the mixture into muffin cups and bake for about 20-25 minutes or until they are cooked through.

15. Low-FODMAP Banana and Blueberry Muffins

Benefits: A sweet and fruity breakfast treat with digestive comfort in mind.

Ingredients:

1 cup gluten-free flour (ensure it's low-FODMAP)

1/2 cup lactose-free milk (e.g., almond milk)

1 ripe banana (ripe but not overripe), mashed

1/2 cup fresh blueberries

1 tablespoon maple syrup (ensure it's low-FODMAP)

Instructions:

Preheat your oven to 350°F (175°C).

In a mixing bowl, combine gluten-free flour, salt, and pepper.

In another bowl, whisk together lactose-free milk, mashed banana, and maple syrup.

Add the wet ingredients to the dry ingredients and mix until just combined.

Gently fold in fresh blueberries.

Spoon the mixture into muffin cups and bake for about 20-25 minutes or until they are cooked through.

Benefits: A nutritious and filling breakfast to energize your day.

Ingredients:

1/4 cup chia seeds

1 cup lactose-free almond milk (or suitable alternative)

1 tablespoon maple syrup (ensure it's low-FODMAP)

Sliced kiwi

Chopped nuts (e.g., almonds or walnuts)

Instructions:

In a bowl, mix chia seeds, lactose-free almond milk, and maple syrup.

Stir well and let the mixture sit in the refrigerator for a few hours or overnight to thicken.

Serve the chia seed breakfast bowl topped with sliced kiwi and chopped nuts.

17. Low-FODMAP Cinnamon French Toast

Benefits: A sweet and comforting breakfast with digestive comfort in mind.

Ingredients:

2 slices of gluten-free bread (ensure it's low-FODMAP)

2 eggs

1/2 cup lactose-free milk (e.g., almond milk)

1/2 teaspoon ground cinnamon

A drizzle of maple syrup (ensure it's low-FODMAP)

Instructions:

In a bowl, whisk together eggs, lactose-free milk, and ground cinnamon.

Dip slices of gluten-free bread into the egg mixture.

Cook the French toast on a griddle.

Drizzle with a touch of maple syrup.

Benefits: A creamy and hearty breakfast without digestive distress.

Ingredients:

1 cup polenta

4 cups lactose-free almond milk (or suitable alternative)

1 tablespoon maple syrup (ensure it's low-FODMAP)

Fresh mixed berries (e.g., strawberries, blueberries)

Instructions:

In a pot, bring lactose-free almond milk to a boil.

Slowly whisk in polenta and reduce heat to low. Stir continuously for about 15-20 minutes until the polenta is thick and creamy.

Stir in maple syrup.

Serve the creamy polenta topped with fresh mixed berries.

19. Low-FODMAP Banana Pancakes

Benefits: A sweet and fluffy breakfast option with digestive comfort in mind.

Ingredients:

1 ripe banana (ripe but not overripe), mashed

1 cup gluten-free pancake mix (ensure it's low-FODMAP)

1/2 cup lactose-free milk (e.g., almond milk)

A drizzle of maple syrup (ensure it's low-FODMAP)

Instructions:

In a bowl, whisk together mashed banana, gluten-free pancake mix, and lactose-free milk.

Cook the pancakes on a griddle.

Drizzle with a touch of maple syrup.

CHAPTER 3: SOUP RECIPES

1. Low-FODMAP Potato Leek Soup

Benefits: A comforting and creamy soup that's gentle on the stomach.

Ingredients:

4 large potatoes, peeled and diced

2 leeks (green tops only), sliced

4 cups low-FODMAP vegetable broth

2 tablespoons garlic-infused olive oil

Salt and pepper to taste

Fresh chives (green tops) for garnish

Instructions:

In a large pot, heat the garlic-infused olive oil over medium heat.

Add sliced leeks and sauté until tender.

Add potatoes, vegetable broth, salt, and pepper.

Simmer until the potatoes are soft.

Blend the soup until smooth.

Garnish with fresh chives and serve.

2. Low-FODMAP Carrot and Ginger Soup

Benefits: A soothing and nutritious soup with digestive benefits.

Ingredients:

6 cups carrots, peeled and chopped

1/4 cup fresh ginger, minced

4 cups low-FODMAP vegetable broth

2 tablespoons garlic-infused olive oil

Salt and pepper to taste

Instructions:

In a large pot, heat the garlic-infused olive oil over medium heat.

Add minced ginger and sauté briefly.

Add chopped carrots, vegetable broth, salt, and pepper.

Simmer until the carrots are tender.

Blend the soup until smooth.

3. Low-FODMAP Tomato Basil Soup

Benefits: A classic soup with a Low-FODMAP twist.

Ingredients:

6 cups canned or fresh diced tomatoes

1 cup fresh basil leaves

2 tablespoons garlic-infused olive oil

Salt and pepper to taste

Instructions:

In a large pot, heat the garlic-infused olive oil over medium heat.

Add diced tomatoes and basil leaves.

Simmer for about 15-20 minutes, stirring occasionally.

Season with salt and pepper.

Blend the soup until smooth.

4. Low-FODMAP Butternut Squash Soup

Benefits: A velvety and hearty soup that's easy to digest.

Ingredients:

1 butternut squash, peeled and diced

2 tablespoons garlic-infused olive oil

4 cups low-FODMAP vegetable broth

Salt and pepper to taste

Fresh chives (green tops) for garnish

Instructions:

In a large pot, heat the garlic-infused olive oil over medium heat.

Add diced butternut squash and vegetable broth.

Simmer until the squash is tender.

Blend the soup until smooth.

Garnish with fresh chives before serving.

5. Low-FODMAP Spinach and Potato Soup

Benefits: A nourishing and satisfying soup with low-FODMAP ingredients.

Ingredients:

4 large potatoes, peeled and diced

4 cups fresh spinach

4 cups low-FODMAP vegetable broth

2 tablespoons garlic-infused olive oil

Salt and pepper to taste

Fresh parsley (green tops) for garnish

Instructions:

In a large pot, heat the garlic-infused olive oil over medium heat.

Add diced potatoes and vegetable broth.

Simmer until the potatoes are soft.

Add fresh spinach and cook until wilted.

Season with salt and pepper.

Garnish with fresh parsley and serve.

6. Low-FODMAP Cucumber and Dill Soup

Benefits: A light and refreshing soup with digestive benefits.

Ingredients:

4 cucumbers, peeled and diced

1/2 cup fresh dill, chopped

4 cups lactose-free yogurt

Salt and pepper to taste

Fresh chives (green tops) for garnish

Instructions:

In a blender, combine diced cucumbers, fresh dill, lactose-free yogurt, salt, and pepper.

Blend until smooth.

Garnish with fresh chives and serve chilled.

7. Low-FODMAP Red Lentil Soup

Benefits: A protein-rich and satisfying soup without digestive distress.

Ingredients:

2 cups red lentils, rinsed

4 cups low-FODMAP vegetable broth

1 cup carrots, peeled and diced

1 cup potatoes, peeled and diced

2 tablespoons garlic-infused olive oil

Cumin, paprika, salt, and pepper to taste

Instructions:

In a large pot, heat the garlic-infused olive oil over medium heat.

Add diced carrots and potatoes, and sauté for a few minutes.

Add red lentils, vegetable broth, and season with cumin, paprika, salt, and pepper.

Simmer until the lentils are tender and the soup has thickened.

8. Low-FODMAP Zucchini Soup

Benefits: A light and flavorful soup with digestive comfort in mind.

Ingredients:

4 zucchinis, diced

4 cups low-FODMAP vegetable broth

2 tablespoons garlic-infused olive oil

Fresh thyme leaves

Salt and pepper to taste

Instructions:

In a large pot, heat the garlic-infused olive oil over medium heat.

Add diced zucchinis and sauté until they start to soften.

Add vegetable broth, fresh thyme leaves, salt, and pepper.

Simmer until the zucchinis are tender.

Blend the soup until smooth.

9. Low-FODMAP Spinach and Coconut Soup

Benefits: A creamy and nutritious soup with low-FODMAP ingredients.

Ingredients:

6 cups fresh spinach

1 can (13.5 oz) coconut milk

2 tablespoons garlic-infused olive oil

Salt and pepper to taste

Fresh cilantro (green tops) for garnish

Instructions:

In a large pot, heat the garlic-infused olive oil over medium heat.

Add fresh spinach and sauté until wilted.

Stir in the coconut milk and simmer for a few minutes.

Season with salt and pepper.

Garnish with fresh cilantro and serve.

Benefits: A traditional Japanese soup with low-FODMAP ingredients.

Ingredients:

4 cups low-FODMAP vegetable broth

1/4 cup miso paste

2 cups firm tofu, cubed

1 cup sliced green tops of scallions

1 sheet nori seaweed, torn into pieces

Instructions:

In a pot, heat the vegetable broth without boiling.

In a separate bowl, dissolve miso pastes in a small amount of warm broth.

Add the miso mixture to the pot and stir.

Add tofu and simmer until heated through.

Serve with sliced green tops of scallions and nori seaweed.

Benefits: A light and flavorful soup with digestive comfort in mind.

Ingredients:

4 cups asparagus, trimmed and chopped

4 cups low-FODMAP vegetable broth

2 tablespoons garlic-infused olive oil

Fresh lemon zest

Salt and pepper to taste

Instructions:

In a large pot, heat the garlic-infused olive oil over medium heat.

Add chopped asparagus and sauté until they start to soften.

Add vegetable broth, fresh lemon zest, salt, and pepper.

Simmer until the asparagus is tender.

Blend the soup until smooth.

12. Low-FODMAP Sweet Potato and Coconut Soup

Benefits: A creamy and sweet soup that's gentle on the stomach.

Ingredients:

2 large sweet potatoes, peeled and diced

1 can (13.5 oz) coconut milk

2 tablespoons garlic-infused olive oil

Fresh cilantro (green tops) for garnish

Salt and pepper to taste

Instructions:

In a large pot, heat the garlic-infused olive oil over medium heat.

Add diced sweet potatoes and sauté for a few minutes.

Stir in the coconut milk and simmer until the sweet potatoes are tender.

Season with salt and pepper.

Garnish with fresh cilantro before serving.

13. Low-FODMAP Spinach and Quinoa Soup

Benefits: A protein-rich and satisfying soup with low-FODMAP ingredients.

Ingredients:

1 cup quinoa

4 cups low-FODMAP vegetable broth

4 cups fresh spinach

2 tablespoons garlic-infused olive oil

Salt and pepper to taste

Instructions:

In a large pot, heat the garlic-infused olive oil over medium heat.

Add quinoa and vegetable broth.

Simmer until the quinoa is cooked and has absorbed the broth.

Stir in fresh spinach and cook until wilted.

Season with salt and pepper.

14. Low-FODMAP Celeriac and Parsnip Soup

Benefits: A nourishing and earthy soup with digestive comfort in mind.

Ingredients:

2 celeriac roots, peeled and diced

2 parsnips, peeled and diced

4 cups low-FODMAP vegetable broth

2 tablespoons garlic-infused olive oil

Fresh thyme leaves

Salt and pepper to taste

Instructions:

In a large pot, heat the garlic-infused olive oil over medium heat.

Add diced celeriac and parsnips, and sauté for a few minutes.

Add vegetable broth, fresh thyme leaves, salt, and pepper.

Simmer until the vegetables are tender.

Blend the soup until smooth.

15. Low-FODMAP Spinach and Lemon Soup

Benefits: A light and zesty soup with digestive benefits.

Ingredients:

6 cups fresh spinach

4 cups low-FODMAP vegetable broth

2 tablespoons garlic-infused olive oil

Zest and juice of one lemon

Salt and pepper to taste

Instructions:

In a large pot, heat the garlic-infused olive oil over medium heat.

Add fresh spinach and sauté until wilted.

Stir in vegetable broth, lemon zest, and lemon juice.

Season with salt and pepper.

Serve with a garnish of extra lemon zest.

Benefits: A hearty and comforting soup that's easy to digest.

Ingredients:

1 small cabbage, shredded

2 cups carrots, peeled and diced

2 cups potatoes, peeled and diced

4 cups low-FODMAP vegetable broth

2 tablespoons garlic-infused olive oil

Fresh dill (green tops) for garnish

Salt and pepper to taste

Instructions:

In a large pot, heat the garlic-infused olive oil over medium heat.

Add shredded cabbage and sauté until it starts to soften.

Stir in carrots, potatoes, vegetable broth, salt, and pepper.

Simmer until the vegetables are tender.

Garnish with fresh dill and serve.

17. Low-FODMAP Kale and White Bean Soup

Benefits: A protein-rich and satisfying soup that's kind to your digestive system.

Ingredients:

6 cups fresh kale, chopped

2 cans (15 oz each) white beans, drained and rinsed

4 cups low-FODMAP vegetable broth

2 tablespoons garlic-infused olive oil

Fresh rosemary (green tops) for garnish

Salt and pepper to taste

Instructions:

In a large pot, heat the garlic-infused olive oil over medium heat.

Add chopped kale and sauté until wilted.

Stir in white beans, vegetable broth, fresh rosemary, salt, and pepper.

Simmer until heated through.

Garnish with fresh rosemary before serving.

18. Low-FODMAP Pumpkin Soup

Benefits: A creamy and warming soup without digestive distress.

Ingredients:

1 can (15 oz) pumpkin puree

4 cups low-FODMAP vegetable broth

2 tablespoons garlic-infused olive oil

Ground nutmeg and cinnamon

Salt and pepper to taste

Fresh chives (green tops) for garnish

Instructions:

In a large pot, heat the garlic-infused olive oil over medium heat.

Add pumpkin puree and vegetable broth.

Season with ground nutmeg, cinnamon, salt, and pepper.

Simmer until heated through.

Garnish with fresh chives before serving

.

19. Low-FODMAP Cauliflower Soup

Benefits: A creamy and savory soup with digestive comfort in mind.

Ingredients:

1 head of cauliflower, chopped

2 cups potatoes, peeled and diced

4 cups low-FODMAP vegetable broth

2 tablespoons garlic-infused olive oil

Fresh thyme leaves

Salt and pepper to taste

Instructions:

In a large pot, heat the garlic-infused olive oil over medium heat.

Add chopped cauliflower, potatoes, and vegetable broth.

Simmer until the vegetables are tender.

Add fresh thyme leaves, salt, and pepper.

Blend the soup until smooth.

CHAPTER 4: SALADS AND SIDES

1. Low-FODMAP Quinoa Salad

Benefits: A protein-packed and nutritious salad that's kind to your digestive system.

Ingredients:

1 cup cooked quinoa

1 cup diced cucumbers; 1 cup diced red bell peppers

1/4 cup chopped fresh parsley (green tops)

2 tablespoons garlic-infused olive oil

1 tablespoon lemon juice

Salt and pepper to taste

Instructions:

In a large bowl, combine cooked quinoa, diced cucumbers, diced red bell peppers, and chopped fresh parsley.

In a separate bowl, whisk together garlic-infused olive oil and lemon juice.

Drizzle the dressing over the salad and toss to combine.

Season with salt and pepper.

2. Low-FODMAP Greek Salad

Benefits: A classic Mediterranean salad with digestive comfort in mind.

Ingredients:

2 cups diced cucumbers

2 cups diced red bell peppers

1 cup chopped fresh parsley (green tops)

1 cup lactose-free feta cheese

Kalamata olives (ensure they are low-FODMAP)

2 tablespoons garlic-infused olive oil

1 tablespoon red wine vinegar

Salt and pepper to taste

Instructions:

In a large bowl, combine diced cucumbers, diced red bell peppers, chopped fresh parsley, lactose-free feta cheese, and Kalamata olives.

In a separate bowl, whisk together garlic-infused olive oil and red wine vinegar.

Drizzle the dressing over the salad and toss to combine.

Season with salt and pepper.

3. Low-FODMAP Tomato and Cucumber Salad

Benefits: A light and refreshing salad with digestive comfort in mind.

Ingredients:

2 cups diced tomatoes

2 cups diced cucumbers

1/4 cup fresh basil leaves

2 tablespoons garlic-infused olive oil

1 tablespoon balsamic vinegar (ensure it's low-FODMAP)

Salt and pepper to taste

Instructions:

In a large bowl, combine diced tomatoes, diced cucumbers, and fresh basil leaves.

In a separate bowl, whisk together garlic-infused olive oil and balsamic vinegar.

Drizzle the dressing over the salad and toss to combine.

Season with salt and pepper.

4. Low-FODMAP Coleslaw

Benefits: A crunchy and creamy coleslaw with digestive comfort in mind.

Ingredients:

4 cups shredded green cabbage

2 cups shredded carrots

1/2 cup lactose-free mayonnaise

2 tablespoons white wine vinegar

1 tablespoon Dijon mustard

1 tablespoon maple syrup (ensure it's low-FODMAP)

Salt and pepper to taste

Instructions:

In a large bowl, combine shredded green cabbage and shredded carrots.

In a separate bowl, whisk together lactose-free mayonnaise, white wine vinegar, Dijon mustard, and maple syrup.

Pour the dressing over the coleslaw and toss to combine.

Season with salt and pepper.

5. Low-FODMAP Potato Salad

Benefits: A classic potato salad with a Low-FODMAP twist.

Ingredients:

4 cups boiled and diced potatoes

1/4 cup diced green tops of scallions

1/4 cup lactose-free mayonnaise

2 tablespoons Dijon mustard

1 tablespoon white wine vinegar

Salt and pepper to taste

Instructions:

In a large bowl, combine diced potatoes and diced green tops of scallions.

In a separate bowl, whisk together lactose-free mayonnaise, Dijon mustard, and white wine vinegar.

Pour the dressing over the potato salad and toss to combine.

Season with salt and pepper.

6. Low-FODMAP Roasted Vegetables

Benefits: A hearty and flavorful side dish with digestive comfort in mind.

Ingredients:

4 cups mixed low-FODMAP vegetables (e.g., zucchini, bell peppers, carrots)

2 tablespoons garlic-infused olive oil

Fresh thyme leaves

Salt and pepper to taste

Instructions:

Preheat your oven to 400°F (200°C).

In a large baking dish, toss mixed low-FODMAP vegetables with garlic-infused olive oil and fresh thyme leaves.

Season with salt and pepper.

Roast in the oven for about 25-30 minutes or until the vegetables are tender and slightly caramelized.

7. Low-FODMAP Spinach and Strawberry Salad

Benefits: A sweet and savory salad with digestive comfort in mind.

Ingredients:

4 cups fresh spinach

1 cup sliced strawberries

1/4 cup chopped pecans

1/4 cup lactose-free feta cheese

2 tablespoons garlic-infused olive oil

1 tablespoon balsamic vinegar (ensure it's low-FODMAP)

Salt and pepper to taste

Instructions:

In a large bowl, combine fresh spinach, sliced strawberries, chopped pecans, and lactose-free feta cheese.

In a separate bowl, whisk together garlic-infused olive oil and balsamic vinegar.

Drizzle the dressing over the salad and toss to combine.

Season with salt and pepper.

8. Low-FODMAP Lemon and Herb Quinoa

Benefits: A zesty and herb-infused quinoa side dish with digestive comfort in mind.

Ingredients:

1 cup cooked quinoa

Zest and juice of one lemon

2 tablespoons fresh basil (green tops), chopped

2 tablespoons fresh mint (green tops), chopped

2 tablespoons garlic-infused olive oil

Salt and pepper to taste

Instructions:

In a large bowl, combine cooked quinoa, lemon zest, lemon juice, chopped fresh basil, and chopped fresh mint.

Drizzle with garlic-infused olive oil.

Season with salt and pepper.

Benefits: A protein-rich and flavorful salad with digestive comfort in mind.

Ingredients:

2 cups cooked and drained chickpeas

1 cup diced cucumbers; 1 cup diced red bell peppers

1/4 cup chopped fresh parsley (green tops)

1/4 cup pitted and sliced black olives (ensure they are low-FODMAP)

2 tablespoons garlic-infused olive oil

1 tablespoon red wine vinegar, Salt and pepper to taste

Instructions:

In a large bowl, combine cooked and drained chickpeas, diced cucumbers, diced red bell peppers, chopped fresh parsley, and sliced black olives.

In a separate bowl, whisk together garlic-infused olive oil and red wine vinegar.

Drizzle the dressing over the salad and toss to combine.

Season with salt and pepper.

10. Low-FODMAP Cucumber and Radish Salad

Benefits: A crisp and refreshing salad with digestive comfort in mind.

Ingredients:

2 cups sliced cucumbers

2 cups sliced radishes

1/4 cup fresh dill (green tops)

2 tablespoons garlic-infused olive oil

1 tablespoon white wine vinegar

Salt and pepper to taste

Instructions:

In a large bowl, combine sliced cucumbers, sliced radishes, and chopped fresh dill.

In a separate bowl, whisk together garlic-infused olive oil and white wine vinegar.

Drizzle the dressing over the salad and toss to combine.

Season with salt and pepper.

11. Low-FODMAP Green Bean Almondine

Benefits: A classic French side dish with digestive comfort in mind.

Ingredients:

4 cups fresh green beans, trimmed

1/4 cup sliced almonds

2 tablespoons garlic-infused olive oil

Zest and juice of one lemon

Salt and pepper to taste

Instructions:

In a pot, blanch the fresh green beans in boiling water for about 3-4 minutes until they are tender-crisp. Drain and immediately place them in ice water to stop the cooking process. Drain again.

In a skillet, toast sliced almonds over medium heat until they are lightly browned.

In the same skillet, heat garlic-infused olive oil over medium heat.

Add blanched green beans and toss to coat.

Sprinkle with lemon zest and lemon juice.

Season with salt and pepper.

12. Low-FODMAP Mashed Potatoes

Benefits: Creamy and comforting mashed potatoes with digestive comfort in mind.

Ingredients:

4 cups peeled and diced potatoes

1/2 cup lactose-free milk (e.g., almond milk)

2 tablespoons garlic-infused olive oil

Salt and pepper to taste

Fresh chives (green tops) for garnish

Instructions:

In a pot, boil the peeled and diced potatoes until they are tender.

Drain and return them to the pot.

Mash the potatoes, gradually adding lactose-free milk and garlic-infused olive oil.

Season with salt and pepper.

Garnish with fresh chives.

13. Low-FODMAP Baked Sweet Potato Fries

Benefits: A crunchy and wholesome side dish with digestive comfort in mind.

Ingredients:

4 cups sweet potatoes, cut into fries

2 tablespoons garlic-infused olive oil

Fresh rosemary (green tops), chopped

Salt and pepper to taste

Instructions:

Preheat your oven to 425°F (220°C).

In a large bowl, toss sweet potato fries with garlic-infused olive oil and chopped fresh rosemary.

Spread the fries in a single layer on a baking sheet.

Bake for about 20-25 minutes, flipping them halfway, until they are crispy and golden.

Benefits: A nutty and flavorful side dish with digestive comfort in mind.

Ingredients:

1 cup cooked brown rice

1/4 cup sliced almonds

2 tablespoons garlic-infused olive oil

Fresh thyme leaves

Salt and pepper to taste

Instructions:

In a skillet, toast sliced almonds over medium heat until they are lightly browned.

In the same skillet, heat garlic-infused olive oil over medium heat.

Add cooked brown rice and toss to coat.

Sprinkle with fresh thyme leaves.

Season with salt and pepper.

15. Low-FODMAP Lemon Asparagus

Benefits: A zesty and vibrant side dish with digestive comfort in mind.

Ingredients:

2 cups fresh asparagus, trimmed

2 tablespoons garlic-infused olive oil

Zest and juice of one lemon

Salt and pepper to taste

Instructions:

In a skillet, heat garlic-infused olive oil over medium heat.

Add fresh asparagus and sauté until they are tender-crisp.

Sprinkle with lemon zest and lemon juice.

Season with salt and pepper.

16. Low-FODMAP Quinoa and Cucumber Salad

Benefits: A light and refreshing side dish with digestive comfort in mind.

Ingredients:

1 cup cooked quinoa

1 cup diced cucumbers

1/4 cup chopped fresh mint (green tops)

2 tablespoons garlic-infused olive oil

1 tablespoon lemon juice

Salt and pepper to taste

Instructions:

In a large bowl, combine cooked quinoa, diced cucumbers, and chopped fresh mint.

In a separate bowl, whisk together garlic-infused olive oil and lemon juice.

Drizzle the dressing over the salad and toss to combine.

Season with salt and pepper.

17. Low-FODMAP Broccoli and Almond Salad

Benefits: A crunchy and nutrient-rich side dish with digestive comfort in mind.

Ingredients:

4 cups steamed and chopped broccoli

1/4 cup sliced almonds

2 tablespoons garlic-infused olive oil

1 tablespoon white wine vinegar

Salt and pepper to taste

Instructions:

In a large bowl, combine steamed and chopped broccoli and sliced almonds.

In a separate bowl, whisk together garlic-infused olive oil and white wine vinegar.

Drizzle the dressing over the salad and toss to combine.

Season with salt and pepper.

18. Low-FODMAP Carrot and Ginger Soup

Benefits: A comforting and flavorful soup with digestive comfort in mind.

Ingredients:

4 cups diced carrots

1 cup diced potatoes

2 tablespoons garlic-infused olive oil

2 tablespoons fresh ginger (green tops), minced

4 cups low-FODMAP vegetable broth

Salt and pepper to taste

Instructions:

In a large pot, heat garlic-infused olive oil over medium heat.

Add diced carrots and diced potatoes, and sauté until slightly softened.

Stir in minced fresh ginger.

Pour in low-FODMAP vegetable broth and simmer until the vegetables are tender.

Blend the soup until smooth.

Season with salt and pepper.

19. Low-FODMAP Zucchini Noodles with Pesto

Benefits: A light and pesto-infused side dish with digestive comfort in mind.

Ingredients:

4 cups spiralized zucchini

1/4 cup lactose-free pesto

Fresh basil leaves (green tops) for garnish

Salt and pepper to taste

Instructions:

In a skillet, heat spiralized zucchini over medium heat until they are heated through.

Toss with lactose-free pesto.

Garnish with fresh basil leaves.

Season with salt and pepper.

20. Low-FODMAP Caprese Salad

Benefits: A classic Italian salad with digestive comfort in mind.

Ingredients:

2 cups sliced tomatoes

1 cup lactose-free mozzarella cheese

Fresh basil leaves (green tops)

2 tablespoons garlic-infused olive oil

Balsamic vinegar glaze (ensure it's low-FODMAP)

Salt and pepper to taste

Instructions:

In a serving dish, layer sliced tomatoes, lactose-free mozzarella cheese, and fresh basil leaves.

Drizzle with garlic-infused olive oil and balsamic vinegar glaze.

Season with salt and pepper.

CHAPTER 5: LUNCH RECIPES

1. Low-FODMAP Quinoa and Vegetable Stir-Fry

Benefits: A quick and flavorful lunch option with digestive comfort in mind.

Ingredients:

1 cup cooked quinoa

1 cup mixed low-FODMAP vegetables (e.g., zucchini, bell peppers, carrots)

2 tablespoons garlic-infused olive oil

2 tablespoons low-sodium soy sauce (ensure it's low-FODMAP)

Fresh cilantro (green tops) for garnish

Salt and pepper to taste

Instructions:

In a wok or skillet, heat garlic-infused olive oil over medium-high heat.

Add mixed low-FODMAP vegetables and stir-fry until they are tender-crisp.

Stir in cooked quinoa and low-sodium soy sauce.

Cook for an additional 2-3 minutes.

Season with salt and pepper.

Garnish with fresh cilantro.

2. Low-FODMAP Greek Salad Wrap

Benefits: A fresh and satisfying wrap with digestive comfort in mind.

Ingredients:

Gluten-free wrap (ensure it's low-FODMAP)

1 cup diced cucumbers

1 cup diced red bell peppers, 1/2 cup lactose-free feta cheese

Kalamata olives (ensure they are low-FODMAP)

Fresh parsley (green tops) for garnish

Low-FODMAP hummus

Salt and pepper to taste

Instructions:

Lay a gluten-free wrap on a clean surface.

Spread a layer of low-FODMAP hummus.

Add diced cucumbers, diced red bell peppers, lactose-free feta cheese, and Kalamata olives.

Season with salt and pepper.

Garnish with fresh parsley.

Roll the wrap and slice in half.

3. Low-FODMAP Caprese Quinoa Salad

Benefits: A light and flavorful salad with digestive comfort in mind.

Ingredients:

1 cup cooked quinoa, 2 cups sliced tomatoes

1 cup lactose-free mozzarella cheese

Fresh basil leaves (green tops)

2 tablespoons garlic-infused olive oil

Balsamic vinegar glaze (ensure it's low-FODMAP)

Salt and pepper to taste

Instructions:

In a large bowl, combine cooked quinoa, sliced tomatoes, lactose-free mozzarella cheese, and fresh basil leaves.

Drizzle with garlic-infused olive oil and balsamic vinegar glaze.

Season with salt and pepper.

4. Low-FODMAP Chickpea and Spinach Salad

Benefits: A protein-rich and nourishing salad with digestive comfort in mind.

Ingredients:

2 cups cooked and drained chickpeas

4 cups fresh spinach

1/2 cup diced red bell peppers

1/4 cup fresh parsley (green tops)

2 tablespoons garlic-infused olive oil

1 tablespoon lemon juice

Salt and pepper to taste

Instructions:

In a large bowl, combine cooked and drained chickpeas, fresh spinach, diced red bell peppers, and fresh parsley.

In a separate bowl, whisk together garlic-infused olive oil and lemon juice.

Drizzle the dressing over the salad and toss to combine.

Season with salt and pepper.

5. Low-FODMAP Tomato and Basil Quiche

Benefits: A savory and satisfying quiche with digestive comfort in mind.

Ingredients:

Gluten-free pie crust (ensure it's low-FODMAP)

4 large eggs

1 cup lactose-free milk (e.g., almond milk)

1 cup sliced tomatoes

1/4 cup fresh basil leaves (green tops)

Salt and pepper to taste

Instructions:

Preheat your oven to 375°F (190°C).

In a bowl, whisk together eggs and lactose-free milk.

Season with salt and pepper.

Arrange sliced tomatoes and fresh basil leaves in the gluten-free pie crust.

Pour the egg mixture over the tomatoes and basil.

Bake for about 30-35 minutes or until the quiche is set and slightly golden.

6. Low-FODMAP Zucchini Noodles with Pesto

Benefits: A light and pesto-infused lunch with digestive comfort in mind.

Ingredients:

4 cups spiralized zucchini

1/4 cup lactose-free pesto

Fresh basil leaves (green tops) for garnish

Salt and pepper to taste

Instructions:

In a skillet, heat spiralized zucchini over medium heat until they are heated through.

Toss with lactose-free pesto.

Garnish with fresh basil leaves.

Season with salt and pepper.

7. Low-FODMAP Cucumber and Radish Sandwich

Benefits: A crisp and refreshing sandwich with digestive comfort in mind.

Ingredients:

Gluten-free bread (ensure it's low-FODMAP)

1 cup sliced cucumbers

1 cup sliced radishes

1/4 cup fresh dill (green tops)

Low-FODMAP mayonnaise

Salt and pepper to taste

Instructions:

Spread a layer of low-FODMAP mayonnaise on two slices of gluten-free bread.

Layer sliced cucumbers and sliced radishes on one slice.

Sprinkle with fresh dill.

Season with salt and pepper.

Top with the second slice of bread and cut the sandwich in half.

8. Low-FODMAP Lemon and Herb Quinoa Salad

Benefits: A zesty and herb-infused salad with digestive comfort in mind.

Ingredients:

1 cup cooked quinoa

Zest and juice of one lemon

2 tablespoons fresh basil (green tops), chopped

2 tablespoons fresh mint (green tops), chopped

2 tablespoons garlic-infused olive oil

Salt and pepper to taste

Instructions:

In a large bowl, combine cooked quinoa, lemon zest, lemon juice, chopped fresh basil, and chopped fresh mint.

Drizzle with garlic-infused olive oil.

Season with salt and pepper.

9. Low-FODMAP Stuffed Bell Peppers

Benefits: A hearty and filling lunch with digestive comfort in mind.

Ingredients:

4 bell peppers (choose low-FODMAP colors)

1 cup cooked quinoa

1 cup mixed low-FODMAP vegetables (e.g., zucchini, carrots)

1/2 cup diced tomatoes

Fresh basil leaves (green tops) for garnish

2 tablespoons garlic-infused olive oil

Salt and pepper to taste

Instructions:

Preheat your oven to 375°F (190°C).

Cut the tops off the bell peppers and remove the seeds.

In a large bowl, combine cooked quinoa, mixed low-FODMAP vegetables, diced tomatoes, and garlic-infused olive oil.

Season with salt and pepper.

Stuff the bell peppers with the quinoa mixture.

Place the stuffed peppers in a baking dish and bake for about 30-35 minutes or until the peppers are tender.

Garnish with fresh basil leaves.

10. Low-FODMAP Mediterranean Rice Bowl

Benefits: A flavorful and well-balanced lunch option with digestive comfort in mind.

Ingredients:

1 cup cooked rice

2 cups mixed low-FODMAP vegetables (e.g., cucumbers, cherry tomatoes)

1/2 cup pitted Kalamata olives (ensure they are low-FODMAP)

1/4 cup feta cheese (ensure it's low-FODMAP)

Fresh parsley (green tops) for garnish

2 tablespoons garlic-infused olive oil

Balsamic vinegar glaze (ensure it's low-FODMAP)

Salt and pepper to taste

Instructions:

In a bowl, combine cooked rice, mixed low-FODMAP vegetables, Kalamata olives, and feta cheese.

Drizzle with garlic-infused olive oil and balsamic vinegar glaze.

Season with salt and pepper.

Garnish with fresh parsley.

Benefits: A savory and filling hash with digestive comfort in mind.

Ingredients:

2 cups diced potatoes

4 cups fresh spinach

1/2 cup diced red bell peppers

1/4 cup fresh chives (green tops)

2 tablespoons garlic-infused olive oil

Salt and pepper to taste

Instructions:

In a skillet, heat garlic-infused olive oil over medium heat.

Add diced potatoes and cook until they are browned and tender.

Stir in fresh spinach, diced red bell peppers, and fresh chives.

Cook until the spinach wilts.

Season with salt and pepper.

12. Low-FODMAP Butternut Squash Soup

Benefits: A creamy and comforting soup with digestive comfort in mind.

Ingredients:

4 cups diced butternut squash

1 cup diced potatoes

2 tablespoons garlic-infused olive oil

4 cups low-FODMAP vegetable broth

Salt and pepper to taste

Instructions:

In a pot, heat garlic-infused olive oil over medium heat.

Add diced butternut squash and potatoes and sauté for a few minutes.

Pour in low-FODMAP vegetable broth and simmer until the vegetables are tender.

Blend the soup until smooth.

Season with salt and pepper.

13. Low-FODMAP Tofu and Vegetable Stir-Fry

Benefits: A protein-packed and satisfying lunch with digestive comfort in mind.

Ingredients:

1 cup cubed firm tofu

1 cup mixed low-FODMAP vegetables (e.g., bok choy, carrots)

2 tablespoons garlic-infused olive oil

2 tablespoons low-sodium soy sauce (ensure it's low-FODMAP)

Sesame seeds (ensure they are low-FODMAP)

Salt and pepper to taste

Instructions:

In a wok or skillet, heat garlic-infused olive oil over medium-high heat.

Add cubed firm tofu and stir-fry until lightly browned.

Add mixed low-FODMAP vegetables and stir-fry until they are tender-crisp.

Stir in low-sodium soy sauce.

Season with sesame seeds, salt, and pepper.

14. Low-FODMAP Cilantro Lime Rice Salad

Benefits: A zesty and aromatic rice salad with digestive comfort in mind.

Ingredients:

1 cup cooked white rice

1/4 cup fresh cilantro (green tops), chopped

Juice of one lime

2 tablespoons garlic-infused olive oil

Salt and pepper to taste

Instructions:

In a large bowl, combine cooked white rice, chopped fresh cilantro, lime juice, and garlic-infused olive oil.

Season with salt and pepper.

15. Low-FODMAP Lentil and Tomato Soup

Benefits: A hearty and protein-rich soup with digestive comfort in mind.

Ingredients:

2 cups cooked and drained lentils

1 cup diced tomatoes

1/2 cup diced carrots

1/4 cup fresh chives (green tops)

4 cups low-FODMAP vegetable broth

2 tablespoons garlic-infused olive oil

Salt and pepper to taste

Instructions:

In a pot, heat garlic-infused olive oil over medium heat.

Add diced tomatoes and diced carrots and sauté for a few minutes.

Stir in cooked and drained lentils and low-FODMAP vegetable broth.

Simmer until the vegetables are tender.

Season with salt and pepper.

Garnish with fresh chives.

CHAPTER 6: DESSERTS RECIPES

1. Low-FODMAP Chocolate Banana Muffins

Benefits: A rich and moist dessert option with digestive comfort in mind.

Ingredients:

1 cup gluten-free flour (ensure it's low-FODMAP)

1/4 cup unsweetened cocoa powder

1/2 cup lactose-free milk (e.g., almond milk)

1 ripe banana (ripe but not overripe), mashed

1/4 cup maple syrup (ensure it's low-FODMAP)

1/4 cup vegetable oil

1 teaspoon baking powder

1/2 teaspoon baking soda

Salt to taste

Instructions:

Preheat your oven to 350°F (175°C).

In a mixing bowl, combine gluten-free flour, cocoa powder, baking powder, baking soda, and a pinch of salt.

In another bowl, whisk together lactose-free milk, mashed banana, maple syrup, and vegetable oil.

Add the wet ingredients to the dry ingredients and mix until just combined.

Spoon the mixture into muffin cups and bake for about 20-25 minutes or until a toothpick comes out clean.

2. Low-FODMAP Berry Parfait

Benefits: A sweet and creamy dessert with digestive comfort in mind.

Ingredients:

1 cup lactose-free Greek yogurt

1/2 cup fresh mixed berries (e.g., strawberries, blueberries)

1 tablespoon maple syrup (ensure it's low-FODMAP)

A sprinkle of gluten-free granola

Instructions:

In a glass, layer lactose-free Greek yogurt, fresh mixed berries, and gluten-free granola.

Drizzle with a touch of maple syrup.

3. Low-FODMAP Rice Pudding

Benefits: A comforting and creamy dessert without digestive distress.

Ingredients:

1 cup cooked white rice

2 cups lactose-free milk (e.g., almond milk)

1/4 cup maple syrup (ensure it's low-FODMAP)

1/2 teaspoon ground cinnamon

1/2 teaspoon vanilla extract

A pinch of salt

Instructions:

In a pot, combine cooked white rice, lactose-free milk, maple syrup, ground cinnamon, and a pinch of salt.

Cook over medium heat, stirring often, until the mixture thickens.

Stir in vanilla extract.

Serve warm or chilled.

4. Low-FODMAP Lemon Sorbet

Benefits: A refreshing and citrusy treat with digestive comfort in mind.

Ingredients:

2 cups freshly squeezed lemon juice

1 cup water

3/4 cup maple syrup (ensure it's low-FODMAP)

Zest of one lemon

Instructions:

In a mixing bowl, whisk together freshly squeezed lemon juice, water, maple syrup, and lemon zest.

Pour the mixture into an ice cream maker and churn according to the manufacturer's instructions.

Transfer the sorbet to a lidded container and freeze until firm.

5. Low-FODMAP Chocolate-Dipped Strawberries

Benefits: A sweet and elegant dessert with digestive comfort in mind.

Ingredients:

Fresh strawberries

1/2 cup dark chocolate chips (ensure they are low-FODMAP)

1 teaspoon coconut oil

Instructions:

Wash and dry fresh strawberries, leaving the green tops on.

In a microwave-safe bowl, melt dark chocolate chips with coconut oil in 20-second intervals, stirring until smooth.

Dip each strawberry into the chocolate mixture.

Place on a parchment paper-lined tray and refrigerate until the chocolate sets.

6. Low-FODMAP Almond and Coconut Bliss Balls

Benefits: A nutty and energy-boosting dessert with digestive comfort in mind.

Ingredients:

1 cup almond meal

1/2 cup shredded coconut

1/4 cup maple syrup (ensure it's low-FODMAP)

2 tablespoons unsweetened cocoa powder

1/4 teaspoon vanilla extract

A pinch of salt

Additional shredded coconut for rolling

Instructions:

In a mixing bowl, combine almond meal, shredded coconut, maple syrup, unsweetened cocoa powder, vanilla extract, and a pinch of salt.

Mix until well combined.

Roll the mixture into bite-sized balls and then roll them in additional shredded coconut.

Refrigerate until firm.

7. Low-FODMAP Pineapple Sorbet

Benefits: A tropical and refreshing dessert with digestive comfort in mind.

Ingredients:

2 cups fresh pineapple chunks

1/2 cup water

1/2 cup maple syrup (ensure it's low-FODMAP)

Juice of one lime

Instructions:

In a blender, combine fresh pineapple chunks, water, maple syrup, and lime juice.

Blend until smooth.

Pour the mixture into an ice cream maker and churn according to the manufacturer's instructions.

Transfer the sorbet to a lidded container and freeze until firm.

8. Low-FODMAP Chocolate Avocado Mousse

Benefits: A creamy and rich chocolate dessert with digestive comfort in mind.

Ingredients:

2 ripe avocados

1/4 cup unsweetened cocoa powder

1/4 cup maple syrup (ensure it's low-FODMAP)

1/2 teaspoon vanilla extract

A pinch of salt

Fresh strawberries for garnish

Instructions:

In a food processor, combine ripe avocados, unsweetened cocoa powder, maple syrup, vanilla extract, and a pinch of salt.

Blend until the mixture is smooth and creamy.

Serve the chocolate avocado mousse with fresh strawberries.

9. Low-FODMAP Rice Crispy Treats

Benefits: A classic and crunchy dessert without digestive distress.

Ingredients:

4 cups rice crisped cereal (ensure it's low-FODMAP)

1/2 cup maple syrup (ensure it's low-FODMAP)

1/2 cup peanut butter (ensure it's low-FODMAP)

1/2 teaspoon vanilla extract

Instructions:

In a large bowl, mix rice crisped cereal.

In a saucepan, heat maple syrup, peanut butter, and vanilla extract over low heat, stirring until well combined.

Pour the peanut butter mixture over the cereal and stir until evenly coated.

Press the mixture into a greased 9x9-inch pan and let it cool and set before cutting into squares.

10. Low-FODMAP Mixed Berry Sorbet

Benefits: A refreshing and antioxidant-packed dessert with digestive comfort in mind.

Ingredients:

2 cups mixed berries (e.g., strawberries, blueberries, raspberries)

1/2 cup water

1/2 cup maple syrup (ensure it's low-FODMAP)

Juice of one lemon

Instructions:

In a blender, combine mixed berries, water, maple syrup, and lemon juice.

Blend until smooth.

Pour the mixture into an ice cream maker and churn according to the manufacturer's instructions.

Transfer the sorbet to a lidded container and freeze until firm.

CHAPTER 7: DINNER RECIPES

1. Low-FODMAP Stuffed Bell Peppers

Benefits: A hearty and filling dinner option with digestive comfort in mind.

Ingredients:

4 bell peppers (choose low-FODMAP colors)

1 cup cooked quinoa

1 cup mixed low-FODMAP vegetables (e.g., zucchini, carrots)

1/2 cup diced tomatoes

Fresh basil leaves (green tops) for garnish

2 tablespoons garlic-infused olive oil

Salt and pepper to taste

Instructions:

Preheat your oven to 375°F (190°C).

Cut the tops off the bell peppers and remove the seeds.

In a large bowl, combine cooked quinoa, mixed low-FODMAP vegetables, diced tomatoes, and garlic-infused olive oil.

Season with salt and pepper.

Stuff the bell peppers with the quinoa mixture.

Place the stuffed peppers in a baking dish and bake for about 30-35 minutes or until the peppers are tender.

Garnish with fresh basil leaves.

2. Low-FODMAP Mediterranean Rice Bowl

Benefits: A flavorful and well-balanced dinner option with digestive comfort in mind.

Ingredients:

1 cup cooked rice

2 cups mixed low-FODMAP vegetables (e.g., cucumbers, cherry tomatoes)

1/2 cup pitted Kalamata olives (ensure they are low-FODMAP)

1/4 cup feta cheese (ensure it's low-FODMAP)

Fresh parsley (green tops) for garnish

2 tablespoons garlic-infused olive oil

Balsamic vinegar glaze (ensure it's low-FODMAP)

Salt and pepper to taste

Instructions:

In a bowl, combine cooked rice, mixed low-FODMAP vegetables, Kalamata olives, and feta cheese.

Drizzle with garlic-infused olive oil and balsamic vinegar glaze.

Season with salt and pepper.

Garnish with fresh parsley.

Benefits: A light and pesto-infused dinner with digestive comfort in mind.

Ingredients:

4 cups spiralized zucchini

1/4 cup lactose-free pesto

Fresh basil leaves (green tops) for garnish

Salt and pepper to taste

Instructions:

In a skillet, heat spiralized zucchini over medium heat until they are heated through.

Toss with lactose-free pesto.

Garnish with fresh basil leaves.

Season with salt and pepper.

4. Low-FODMAP Greek Salad Wrap

Benefits: A fresh and satisfying wrap with digestive comfort in mind.

Ingredients:

Gluten-free wrap (ensure it's low-FODMAP)

1 cup diced cucumbers; 1 cup diced red bell peppers

1/2 cup lactose-free feta cheese

Kalamata olives (ensure they are low-FODMAP)

Fresh parsley (green tops) for garnish

Low-FODMAP hummus

Salt and pepper to taste

Instructions:

Lay a gluten-free wrap on a clean surface.

Spread a layer of low-FODMAP hummus.

Add diced cucumbers, diced red bell peppers, lactose-free feta cheese, and Kalamata olives.

Season with salt and pepper.

Garnish with fresh parsley.

Roll the wrap and slice in half.

5. Low-FODMAP Tomato and Basil Quiche

Benefits: A savory and satisfying quiche with digestive comfort in mind.

Ingredients:

Gluten-free pie crust (ensure it's low-FODMAP)

4 large eggs

1 cup lactose-free milk (e.g., almond milk)

1 cup sliced tomatoes

1/4 cup fresh basil leaves (green tops)

Salt and pepper to taste

Instructions:

Preheat your oven to 375°F (190°C).

In a bowl, whisk together eggs and lactose-free milk.

Season with salt and pepper.

Arrange sliced tomatoes and fresh basil leaves in the gluten-free pie crust.

Pour the egg mixture over the tomatoes and basil.

Bake for about 30-35 minutes or until the quiche is set and slightly golden.

Benefits: A protein-packed and satisfying dinner with digestive comfort in mind.

Ingredients:

1 cup cubed firm tofu

1 cup mixed low-FODMAP vegetables (e.g., bok choy, carrots)

2 tablespoons garlic-infused olive oil

2 tablespoons low-sodium soy sauce (ensure it's low-FODMAP)

Sesame seeds (ensure they are low-FODMAP)

Salt and pepper to taste

Instructions:

In a wok or skillet, heat garlic-infused olive oil over medium-high heat.

Add cubed firm tofu and stir-fry until lightly browned.

Add mixed low-FODMAP vegetables and stir-fry until they are tender-crisp.

Stir in low-sodium soy sauce.

Season with sesame seeds, salt, and pepper.

Benefits: A crisp and refreshing salad with digestive comfort in mind.

Ingredients:

2 cups sliced cucumbers

1 cup sliced radishes

1/4 cup fresh dill (green tops)

2 tablespoons garlic-infused olive oil

1 tablespoon white wine vinegar

Salt and pepper to taste

Instructions:

In a large bowl, combine sliced cucumbers, sliced radishes, and fresh dill.

In a separate bowl, whisk together garlic-infused olive oil and white wine vinegar.

Drizzle the dressing over the salad and toss to combine.

Season with salt and pepper.

8. Low-FODMAP Mexican Quinoa Bowl

Benefits: A flavorful and protein-rich dinner option with digestive comfort in mind.

Ingredients:

1 cup cooked quinoa

1 cup mixed low-FODMAP vegetables (e.g., bell peppers, corn)

1/2 cup cooked black beans

1/4 cup diced tomatoes

2 tablespoons fresh cilantro (green tops), chopped

2 tablespoons garlic-infused olive oil

1 tablespoon low-sodium taco seasoning (ensure it's low-FODMAP)

Salt and pepper to taste

Instructions:

In a bowl, combine cooked quinoa, mixed low-FODMAP vegetables, cooked black beans, diced tomatoes, and fresh cilantro.

In a separate bowl, mix garlic-infused olive oil and low-sodium taco seasoning.

Drizzle the dressing over the quinoa mixture.

Season with salt and pepper.

9. Low-FODMAP Eggplant Parmesan

Benefits: A comforting and cheesy dish with digestive comfort in mind.

Ingredients:

2 small eggplants

1 cup gluten-free breadcrumbs (ensure they're low-FODMAP)

1/4 cup grated Parmesan cheese (ensure it's low-FODMAP)

1 cup lactose-free marinara sauce

1 cup lactose-free mozzarella cheese

2 tablespoons garlic-infused olive oil

Fresh basil leaves (green tops) for garnish

Salt and pepper to taste

Instructions:

Preheat your oven to 375°F (190°C).

Slice the eggplants into rounds.

In a bowl, combine gluten-free breadcrumbs and grated Parmesan cheese.

Dip the eggplant rounds into the breadcrumb mixture to coat.

In a skillet, heat garlic-infused olive oil over medium heat.

Sear the eggplant rounds until they are browned.

In a baking dish, layer eggplant rounds, lactose-free marinara sauce, and lactose-free mozzarella cheese.

Repeat the layers.

Bake for about 25-30 minutes or until the cheese is bubbly and golden.

Garnish with fresh basil leaves.

10. Low-FODMAP Lemon and Herb Quinoa Salad

Benefits: A zesty and herb-infused salad with digestive comfort in mind.

Ingredients:

1 cup cooked quinoa

Zest and juice of one lemon

2 tablespoons fresh basil (green tops), chopped

2 tablespoons fresh mint (green tops), chopped

2 tablespoons garlic-infused olive oil

Salt and pepper to taste

Instructions:

In a large bowl, combine cooked quinoa, lemon zest, lemon juice, chopped fresh basil, and chopped fresh mint.

Drizzle with garlic-infused olive oil.

Season with salt and pepper.

11. Low-FODMAP Spinach and Potato Hash

Benefits: A savory and filling hash with digestive comfort in mind.

Ingredients:

2 cups diced potatoes

4 cups fresh spinach

1/2 cup diced red bell peppers

1/4 cup fresh chives (green tops)

2 tablespoons garlic-infused olive oil

Salt and pepper to taste

Instructions:

In a skillet, heat garlic-infused olive oil over medium heat.

Add diced potatoes and cook until they are browned and tender.

Stir in fresh spinach, diced red bell peppers, and fresh chives.

Cook until the spinach wilts.

Season with salt and pepper.

12. Low-FODMAP Butternut Squash Soup

Benefits: A creamy and comforting soup with digestive comfort in mind.

Ingredients:

4 cups diced butternut squash

1 cup diced potatoes

2 tablespoons garlic-infused olive oil

4 cups low-FODMAP vegetable broth

Salt and pepper to taste

Instructions:

In a pot, heat garlic-infused olive oil over medium heat.

Add diced butternut squash and potatoes and sauté for a few minutes.

Pour in low-FODMAP vegetable broth and simmer until the vegetables are tender.

Blend the soup until smooth.

Season with salt and pepper.

13. Low-FODMAP Lentil and Tomato Soup

Benefits: A hearty and protein-rich soup with digestive comfort in mind.

Ingredients:

2 cups cooked and drained lentils

1 cup diced tomatoes

1/2 cup diced carrots

1/4 cup fresh chives (green tops)

4 cups low-FODMAP vegetable broth

2 tablespoons garlic-infused olive oil

Salt and pepper to taste

Instructions:

In a pot, heat garlic-infused olive oil over medium heat.

Add diced tomatoes and diced carrots and sauté for a few minutes.

Stir in cooked and drained lentils and low-FODMAP vegetable broth.

Simmer until the vegetables are tender.

Season with salt and pepper.

Garnish with fresh chives.

14. Low-FODMAP Cilantro Lime Rice Salad

Benefits: A zesty and aromatic rice salad with digestive comfort in mind.

Ingredients:

1 cup cooked white rice

1/4 cup fresh cilantro (green tops), chopped

Juice of one lime

2 tablespoons garlic-infused olive oil

Salt and pepper to taste

Instructions:

In a large bowl, combine cooked white rice, chopped fresh cilantro, lime juice, and garlic-infused olive oil.

Season with salt and pepper.

15. Low-FODMAP Mexican Stuffed Peppers

Benefits: A flavorful and protein-rich dinner with digestive comfort in mind.

Ingredients:

4 bell peppers (choose low-FODMAP colors)

1 cup cooked rice

1 cup cooked and drained black beans

1/2 cup diced tomatoes

1/2 cup diced red bell peppers

2 tablespoons garlic-infused olive oil

1 tablespoon low-sodium taco seasoning (ensure it's low-FODMAP)

Salt and pepper to taste

Instructions:

Preheat your oven to 375°F (190°C).

Cut the tops off the bell peppers and remove the seeds.

In a large bowl, combine cooked rice, cooked and drained black beans, diced tomatoes, diced red bell peppers, garlic-infused olive oil, and low-sodium taco seasoning.

Season with salt and pepper.

Stuff the bell peppers with the mixture.

Place the stuffed peppers in a baking dish and bake for about 30-35 minutes or until the peppers are tender.

CONCLUSION

This Low-FODMAP Vegetarian Cookbook is not merely a collection of recipes; it is a roadmap to a healthier and more comfortable digestive journey. By adopting the principles of the Low-FODMAP diet while savoring the flavors of plant-based cuisine, you are starting a path to wellness that is both satisfying and gentle on your digestive system.

The benefits of this cookbook are abundant. It empowers you to make informed choices, embrace a nourishing diet, and explore the world of delicious low-FODMAP vegetarian dishes. Whether you're new to the Low-FODMAP diet or have been following it for a while, you'll find these recipes to be a source of culinary inspiration and a guide to maintaining digestive comfort.

If you are seeking to embark on a Low-FODMAP journey, this cookbook serves as a trustworthy companion. You'll discover a diverse array of recipes that encompass breakfast, lunch, dinner, soups, salads, sides, and even desserts, all thoughtfully crafted to ensure your dietary needs are met without sacrificing flavor. With each recipe, you can indulge in dishes that not only support your digestive health but also delight your taste buds.

Additionally, the wealth of information provided on FODMAPs, the Low-FODMAP diet, and its impact on digestive discomfort is designed to empower you with knowledge. This knowledge equips you to make informed choices and create a sustainable, health-focused approach to eating that can lead to long-lasting well-being.

By using this cookbook, you're making a commitment to prioritize your health without compromising on taste. Each recipe is carefully crafted to exclude high-FODMAP ingredients while maintaining the deliciousness of your meals. With this cookbook in hand, you can embark on a Low-FODMAP journey with confidence, experiencing the benefits of improved digestive comfort, reduced discomfort, and a renewed sense of vitality.

MEAL PLANNER
WEEK 1

Meal Planner

Date:

Monday	Tuesday	Wednesday
BREAKFAST	BREAKFAST	BREAKFAST
LUNCH	LUNCH	LUNCH
DINNER	DINNER	DINNER
DESSERTS	DESSERTS	DESSERTS

Thursday	Friday	Saturday
BREAKFAST	BREAKFAST	BREAKFAST
LUNCH	LUNCH	LUNCH
DINNER	DINNER	DINNER
DESSERTS	DESSERTS	DESSERTS

Sunday	NOTES:
BREAKFAST	
LUNCH	
DINNER	
DESSERTS	

WEEK-2

Meal Planner

Date:

Monday
BREAKFAST

LUNCH

DINNER

DESSERTS

Tuesday
BREAKFAST

LUNCH

DINNER

DESSERTS

Wednesday
BREAKFAST

LUNCH

DINNER

DESSERTS

Thursday
BREAKFAST

LUNCH

DINNER

DESSERTS

Friday
BREAKFAST

LUNCH

DINNER

DESSERTS

Saturday
BREAKFAST

LUNCH

DINNER

DESSERTS

Sunday
BREAKFAST

LUNCH

DINNER

DESSERTS

NOTES:

WEEK-3

Meal Planner

Date:

Monday	Tuesday	Wednesday
BREAKFAST	BREAKFAST	BREAKFAST
LUNCH	LUNCH	LUNCH
DINNER	DINNER	DINNER
DESSERTS	DESSERTS	DESSERTS

Thursday	Friday	Saturday
BREAKFAST	BREAKFAST	BREAKFAST
LUNCH	LUNCH	LUNCH
DINNER	DINNER	DINNER
DESSERTS	DESSERTS	DESSERTS

Sunday	NOTES:
BREAKFAST	
LUNCH	
DINNER	
DESSERTS	

WEEK-4

Meal Planner

Date:

Monday
BREAKFAST

LUNCH

DINNER

DESSERTS

Tuesday
BREAKFAST

LUNCH

DINNER

DESSERTS

Wednesday
BREAKFAST

LUNCH

DINNER

DESSERTS

Thursday
BREAKFAST

LUNCH

DINNER

DESSERTS

Friday
BREAKFAST

LUNCH

DINNER

DESSERTS

Saturday
BREAKFAST

LUNCH

DINNER

DESSERTS

Sunday
BREAKFAST

LUNCH

DINNER

DESSERTS

NOTES:

Made in United States
Troutdale, OR
02/09/2024

17545161R00076